Heart Disease Cookbook

35+ Tasty Heart Healthy and Low Sodium Recipes

copyright © 2021 Larry Jamesonn

All rights reserved No part of this book may be reproduced, or stored in a retrieval system, or transmitted in any form or by any means, electronic, mechanical, photocopying, recording, or otherwise, without express written permission of the publisher.

Disclaimer

By reading this disclaimer, you are accepting the terms of the disclaimer in full. If you disagree with this disclaimer, please do not read the guide.

All of the content within this guide is provided for informational and educational purposes only, and should not be accepted as independent medical or other professional advice. The author is not a doctor, physician, nurse, mental health provider, or registered nutritionist/dietician. Therefore, using and reading this guide does not establish any form of a physician-patient relationship.

Always consult with a physician or another qualified health provider with any issues or questions you might have regarding any sort of medical condition. Do not ever disregard any qualified professional medical advice or delay seeking that advice because of anything you have read in this guide. The information in this guide is not intended to be any sort of medical advice and should not be used in lieu of any medical advice by a licensed and qualified medical professional.

The information in this guide has been compiled from a variety of known sources. However, the author cannot attest to or guarantee the accuracy of each source and thus should not be held liable for any errors or omissions.

You acknowledge that the publisher of this guide will not be held liable for any loss or damage of any kind incurred as a result of this guide or the reliance on any information provided within this guide. You acknowledge and agree that you assume all risk and responsibility for any action you undertake in response to the information in this guide.

Using this guide does not guarantee any particular result (e.g., weight loss or a cure). By reading this guide, you acknowledge that there are no guarantees to any specific outcome or results you can expect.

All product names, diet plans, or names used in this guide are for identification purposes only and are the property of their respective owners. The use of these names does not imply endorsement. All other trademarks cited herein are the property of their respective owners.

Where applicable, this guide is not intended to be a substitute for the original work of this diet plan and is, at most, a supplement to the original work for this diet plan and never a direct substitute. This guide is a personal expression of the facts of that diet plan.

Where applicable, persons shown in the cover images are stock photography models and the publisher has obtained the rights to use the images through license agreements with third-party stock image companies.

Table of Contents

Introduction	**8**
What Is Heart Disease?	**10**
Causes of Heart Disease	11
Symptoms of Heart Disease	13
Preventing Heart Disease	14
Foods to Eat for a Heart-Healthy Diet	**16**
Fruits and Vegetables	16
Whole Grains	17
Healthy Fats	17
Proteins	18
Dairy	19
Beverages	19
Herbs and Spices	19
Additional Tips	20
Foods to Avoid for a Heart-Healthy Diet	**21**
Processed and Red Meats	21
Trans Fats and Saturated Fats	22
High-Sodium Foods	22
Sugary Foods and Beverages	23
Refined Carbohydrates	23
Alcohol	23
Some Dairy Products	24
Foods High in Added Sugars	24
Sample 7-Day Meal Plan for a Healthier Heart	**25**
Recipe List	**29**
Apple and Onion Mix	30
Shrimp and Egg Fried Rice	31
Grilled Eggplant	33
Mixed Vegetable Roast with Lemon Zest	34

Pepper Ginger Beef Stir-Fry	36
Salmon and Asparagus	38
Baked Salmon	40
Roasted Veggies	42
Trout Scrambler	43
Mixed Veggie Fried Rice	45
Arugula and Mushroom Salad	46
Cypriot Cheese and Greens Salad with Pesto Dressing	47
Macrobiotic Bowl Medley	49
Broccoli-Kale with Avocado Toppings Rice Bowl	51
Stir-fry Broccoli, Onions, and Carrots	52
Banana Bread	53
Butternut Squash with Turmeric Soup	55
Cheddar Turkey Deviled Egg	57
Go Green Blueberries	59
Spinach and Kale Blend	60
Energy Boost Smoothie	61
Green and Berry Smoothie	62
Almond Surf Smoothie	63
Toasted Almond Banana Mix	64
Berry Blast English Muffin	65
Berry Blast Oats	66
Apple Cinnamon Smash Oatmeal	67
Energizing Oatmeal	68
Quinoa-Based Oriental Salad	69
Hearty Chicken Salad with Pasta	71
Heart Helping Cobb	73
Grenade Salad	75
Chicken Breast Delight	77
Sun Crust Turkey Cuts	78
Turkish Meatballs in Marinara	80

Hot, Hot, Hot Salmon	82
Taste of Mediterranean	83
Avocado and Tomato Whole Wheat Pasta Salad	85
Lentil Vegetable Soup	86
Grilled Vegetable and Hummus Wrap	88
Apple Cinnamon Oatmeal	89
Turkey and Veggie Stuffed Peppers	90
Conclusion	**92**
FAQ	**95**
References and Helpful Links	**98**

Introduction

Navigating the path to heart-healthy eating can often seem like walking through a maze—complex and full of uncertainties. Yet, it's a journey that holds the promise of a healthier, more vibrant life. This guide crafted to demystify this path, offering a collection of recipes that are as good for your heart as they are for your taste buds. It's an invitation to transform your diet without sacrificing the joy of eating.

In a world where heart disease continues to be a leading health issue, affecting millions each year, the importance of diet cannot be overstated. But finding reliable, straightforward advice on cooking heart-healthy meals can be challenging. This is where this guide comes into play—a beacon for those seeking not just guidance, but also inspiration in their daily meals.

This guide is more than a simple collection of recipes; it's a comprehensive resource designed by a team of nutrition experts and culinary professionals. They have poured their knowledge and passion into creating dishes that blend nutritional science with culinary art. From breakfasts that energize to dinners that satisfy, these recipes prove that heart-healthy meals can also be mouth wateringly delicious.

The joy of sitting down to a meal that not only tastes fantastic but also contributes to your health is immeasurable. With ths guide, this becomes an everyday reality. Each recipe is carefully crafted to ensure that it supports heart health, using ingredients that are known for their positive impact on cardiovascular wellness. This guide empowers you to make informed choices about what you eat, providing peace of mind and a sense of well-being with every dish.

In this guide, we will talk about the following;

- What is Heart Disease?
- Causes, Symptoms, and How to Prevent Heart Disease
- Foods to Eat and To Avoid for A Heart-Healthy Diet
- 7-Day Sample Meal Plan
- Sample Recipes

Start your heart-healthy culinary adventure today. Each recipe represents a step toward a healthier heart and a testament to the belief that nourishing meals can and should be delicious. Whether you are directly affected by heart disease or aiming to prevent it, this guide is your ally, ready to show you that eating for your heart can also mean eating for pleasure.

What Is Heart Disease?

Heart disease, encompassing a range of conditions such as coronary artery disease, heart rhythm problems, and congenital heart defects, remains one of the most significant health challenges globally.

Its impact on health is profound, often leading to serious complications like heart attacks, strokes, and chronic heart failure, which significantly affect life quality and longevity. The root causes are multifaceted, including lifestyle factors, genetic predisposition, and other risk factors like high blood pressure, smoking, and diabetes.

Diet plays a pivotal role in the management and prevention of heart disease. The connection between what we eat and heart health is unmistakable; diets high in saturated fats, trans fats, and sodium can exacerbate risks, whereas those rich in fruits, vegetables, whole grains, and lean proteins can mitigate them.

A heart-healthy diet can help lower blood pressure, improve cholesterol levels, reduce inflammation, and maintain a healthy weight—key factors in reducing the risk of heart disease. By making informed dietary choices, individuals have the power to influence their heart health positively, highlighting the importance of diet not just in managing existing heart disease but in preventing its onset.

Causes of Heart Disease

Heart disease can result from a variety of factors, many of which are interconnected. Some of the primary causes and risk factors include:

- *Unhealthy Diet*: Consuming excessive amounts of saturated fats, trans fats, sodium, and sugars can lead to conditions that increase the risk of heart disease, such as high blood pressure, high cholesterol, and obesity.
- *Physical Inactivity*: A lack of regular exercise is associated with a higher risk of heart disease, as physical activity helps control weight, and reduces chances of developing conditions that strain the heart, like high blood pressure and type 2 diabetes.
- *Obesity*: Being overweight or obese increases the stress on the heart and is a risk factor for heart disease. Obesity is also linked to other risk factors, such as high blood cholesterol and triglyceride levels, and high blood pressure.
- *Smoking and Use of Tobacco*: Smoking and tobacco use significantly increase the risk of heart disease. Chemicals in tobacco damage the heart and blood

vessels, leading to the narrowing of the arteries (atherosclerosis), which can cause heart attacks.
- *Excessive Alcohol Consumption*: Drinking too much alcohol can raise blood pressure, increase cardiomyopathy, and contribute to other heart disease risk factors like obesity.
- *High Blood Pressure (Hypertension)*: High blood pressure puts additional force against the artery walls, which can damage them over time, increasing the risk of heart disease.
- *High Cholesterol*: High levels of bad cholesterol (LDL) can lead to the buildup of plaques in the arteries, reducing or blocking blood flow to the heart.
- *Diabetes*: Diabetes increases the risk of heart disease significantly, as it's associated with high blood sugar levels that can damage blood vessels and the nerves that control the heart.
- *Age*: Aging increases your risk of damaged and narrowed arteries and weakened or thickened heart muscle.
- *Family History of Heart Disease*: If heart disease runs in the family, you may be at higher risk, especially if a close relative develops heart disease at an early age.
- *Stress*: Long-term stress and poor reactions to stress can increase the risk of hypertension, heart attacks, and other heart-related issues.

- ***Poor Sleep Health***: Sleep apnea and other sleep disorders can increase the risk of heart disease.

While some risk factors like age and family history cannot be changed, many of the causes of heart disease can be managed or prevented through lifestyle changes and, when necessary, medication.

Symptoms of Heart Disease

Early detection of heart disease is crucial for prompt treatment and reducing the risk of complications. Some common symptoms of heart disease include:

- Chest pain or discomfort (angina)
- Shortness of breath
- Pain, numbness, and/or tingling in the arms or legs
- Indigestion, nausea, or vomiting
- Dizziness or lightheadedness
- Fatigue or weakness

If you experience any of these symptoms, it's important to consult your doctor for a proper diagnosis and treatment plan. It's also essential to be aware of any specific risk factors that may increase your chances of developing heart disease.

Preventing Heart Disease

Preventing heart disease involves making healthy lifestyle choices and managing underlying medical conditions. Here are some ways to reduce your risk of heart disease:

- *Quit smoking*: Smoking is a major cause of heart disease, so quitting can significantly decrease your risk.
- *Exercise regularly*: Regular physical activity can improve cardiovascular health and reduce the risk of heart disease.
- *Eat a healthy diet*: A diet rich in fruits, vegetables, whole grains, and lean proteins can help maintain a healthy weight and reduce the risk of heart disease.
- *Manage medical conditions*: If you have high blood pressure, high cholesterol, or diabetes, it's important to work with your doctor to manage these conditions and reduce their impact on your heart health.
- *Reduce stress*: Chronic stress can have a negative impact on your heart health. Finding healthy ways to manage stress, such as exercise, meditation, or therapy, can help improve cardiovascular health.
- *Limit alcohol consumption*: Excessive alcohol intake can lead to high blood pressure and increase the risk of heart disease. It's important to limit alcohol consumption to moderate levels (one drink per day for women and two drinks per day for men).

By implementing these lifestyle changes, you can greatly reduce your risk of developing heart disease. It's also important to keep up with regular check-ups and screenings, as early detection and treatment can significantly improve outcomes for those at risk of heart disease. Additionally, staying educated about heart health and making informed decisions about your diet, exercise habits, and medical care can go a long way in preventing heart disease.

Foods to Eat for a Heart-Healthy Diet

A heart-healthy diet is crucial for maintaining cardiovascular health and preventing heart disease. By focusing on a variety of whole, unprocessed foods, you can ensure your body receives the essential nutrients it needs. Below is an expanded look at the best food groups to include in a heart-healthy diet:

Fruits and Vegetables

- *Leafy Green Vegetables*: Spinach, kale, and collard greens are powerhouses of vitamins, minerals, and antioxidants, all of which support heart health. They are high in vitamin K, which helps protect your arteries and promote proper blood clotting. Additionally, they're a great source of dietary nitrates, which have been shown to reduce blood pressure, decrease arterial stiffness, and improve the function of cells lining the blood vessels.
- *Whole Fruits*: Berries such as strawberries, blueberries, raspberries, and blackberries are rich in important nutrients and antioxidants like anthocyanins,

which can protect against oxidative stress and inflammation that contribute to heart disease. Oranges, apples, and pears are also excellent choices, offering high fiber content, which helps lower cholesterol levels and improves heart health.

Whole Grains

- *Oats and Oatmeal*: A standout for their high soluble fiber content, particularly beta-glucan, oats can significantly lower cholesterol levels and thus reduce the risk of heart disease. Regular consumption of oats is associated with lower blood pressure and a reduced risk of coronary artery disease.
- *Whole Wheat, Brown Rice, Barley, and Quinoa*: These grains are good sources of fiber, vitamins, minerals, and phytochemicals that work together to support heart health. They help improve blood cholesterol levels and protect against high blood pressure.

Healthy Fats

- *Avocados*: Rich in monounsaturated fats, avocados can help reduce bad LDL cholesterol levels while raising good HDL cholesterol. They're also a good source of potassium, a nutrient that's essential in managing blood pressure.

- *Nuts and Seeds*: Walnuts, almonds, flaxseeds, and chia seeds not only offer heart-healthy fats but also fiber and omega-3 fatty acids. Regular consumption of these nuts and seeds has been linked to a reduced risk of heart disease, lower levels of inflammation, and improved arterial function.
- *Olive Oil*: A key component of the Mediterranean diet, olive oil is celebrated for its monounsaturated fats and antioxidants, which can diminish the risk of heart disease by improving cholesterol levels and reducing inflammation.

Proteins

- *Fatty Fish*: Salmon, mackerel, sardines, and trout are excellent sources of omega-3 fatty acids, which have been shown to lower the risk of arrhythmias (irregular heartbeats), decrease triglyceride levels, and slightly lower blood pressure.
- *Legumes*: Beans, lentils, and peas are fantastic plant-based protein sources that offer high amounts of fiber, vitamins, and minerals. Including legumes in your diet can help lower blood pressure and improve other cardiovascular risk factors.
- *Lean Poultry*: Opting for skinless chicken or turkey provides a high-quality protein with less saturated fat compared to red meat, making it a better choice for heart health.

Dairy

Low-Fat or Non-Fat Dairy Products: Incorporating milk, yogurt, and cheese in their low-fat or non-fat versions can provide essential nutrients such as calcium, potassium, and vitamin D, without the added saturated fat that can contribute to heart disease.

Beverages

- *Water*: Adequate hydration is vital for overall health, including heart health. Water assists in the maintenance of blood volume and the transport of nutrients and oxygen throughout your body.
- *Green Tea*: Rich in antioxidants called catechins, green tea can help improve blood lipid levels and reduce inflammation. Drinking green tea has been associated with a lower risk of heart disease and stroke.

Herbs and Spices

- *Turmeric, Garlic, Ginger*: These are known for their anti-inflammatory and antioxidant properties. Turmeric contains curcumin, which can improve endothelial function. Garlic has been shown to lower blood pressure and cholesterol levels. Ginger aids in lowering blood pressure and has anti-inflammatory effects.

- *Fresh Herbs*: Adding herbs like parsley, cilantro, and basil can enhance the flavor of dishes without the need for added salt, helping to manage blood pressure.

Additional Tips

1. *Limit Trans and Saturated Fats*: Opting for lean meats and plant-based sources of protein, while avoiding fried and processed foods, can help reduce intake of unhealthy fats.
2. *Reduce Sodium Intake*: Choosing fresh over processed foods and seasoning with herbs and spices instead of salt can significantly lower sodium intake, which is crucial for managing blood pressure.
3. *Minimize Added Sugars*: Consuming too much sugar can lead to weight gain and increase the risk of heart disease. Focus on whole foods and limit processed foods and beverages high in added sugars.

Remember, achieving a heart-healthy diet is about balance and variety. Incorporating a wide range of nutritious foods while limiting the intake of unhealthy fats, added sugars, and sodium is key. Alongside dietary changes, regular physical activity, and consulting with healthcare providers for personalized advice are also important steps to maintain heart health.

Foods to Avoid for a Heart-Healthy Diet

Adopting a heart-healthy diet involves being mindful of not just what to include, but also what foods to limit or avoid. Certain foods can contribute to increased risk factors for heart disease, including elevated cholesterol levels, high blood pressure, and weight gain. Here's an expanded look into the types of foods best reduced or avoided for heart health:

Processed and Red Meats

- *Processed Meats*: Items like sausages, hot dogs, and bacon are typically high in saturated fats, sodium, and preservatives. Regular consumption is linked to an increased risk of cardiovascular diseases and hypertension due to their high content of unhealthy fats and salt.
- *Red Meats*: It's advisable to limit the intake of beef, pork, and lamb. These meats contain higher amounts of saturated fats compared to their white meat counterparts. Saturated fats can raise the level of bad

cholesterol (LDL) in your blood, contributing to the buildup of plaque in your arteries.

Trans Fats and Saturated Fats

- *Trans Fats*: Often found in fried foods, commercially baked goods (like pastries and cookies), and any products made with partially hydrogenated oils, trans fats are especially harmful because they raise LDL cholesterol and lower HDL (good) cholesterol, increasing the risk of heart disease.
- *Saturated Fats*: Present in full-fat dairy products, butter, and high-fat cuts of meat. Consuming too much saturated fat can increase total cholesterol and LDL cholesterol levels. Opting for low-fat or fat-free versions can help reduce these risks.

High-Sodium Foods

- *Processed Foods*: Items like canned soups, frozen dinners, and processed snacks often contain excessive sodium, which can lead to hypertension, a major risk factor for heart disease.
- *Fast Food*: Typically laden with sodium, saturated fats, and calories, fast food can contribute significantly to heart disease risk factors, including obesity and high blood pressure.

Sugary Foods and Beverages

- *Sugary Drinks*: Beverages like soda, fruit juices with added sugars, and energy drinks are high in calories and sugar but low in nutritional value. They can contribute to weight gain, inflammation, and elevated triglyceride levels, all of which are risk factors for heart disease.
- *Candy and Sweets*: These are often high in added sugars and may include unhealthy fats, contributing to poor heart health, obesity, and diabetes.

Refined Carbohydrates

- *White Bread, Pasta, and Rice*: These refined grains have been stripped of their fiber and nutrients, leading to rapid spikes in blood sugar and insulin levels, which over time can lead to diabetes and heart disease.
- *Pastries and Other Baked Goods*: Typically high in sugar, saturated fats, and refined flour, these foods can contribute to weight gain and increased LDL cholesterol levels.

Alcohol

Excessive Alcohol Consumption: While moderate alcohol consumption might have some heart benefits, excessive drinking can raise blood pressure, cause irregular heartbeats, and lead to weight gain. Limiting intake is key to managing heart health.

Some Dairy Products

High-Fat Dairy Products: Cream, full-fat cheese, and butter are high in saturated fats. Choosing low-fat or non-fat dairy options can help manage cholesterol levels.

Foods High in Added Sugars

Processed Snacks and Desserts: Many cookies, cakes, ice creams, and candy bars are loaded with added sugars and unhealthy fats, offering little nutritional value and posing risks to heart health.

In general, prioritizing a diet focused on whole, minimally processed foods and rich in fruits, vegetables, whole grains, lean proteins, and healthy fats can significantly contribute to maintaining heart health. It's important to consult with healthcare professionals or dietitians to create a diet plan that addresses your specific health needs and goals.

Sample 7-Day Meal Plan for a Healthier Heart

By opting for our Sample 7-Day Meal Plan for a Healthier Heart, you're making a choice to nurture your heart with the attention it needs. Each meal in the plan is crafted to bolster your heart's health, blending tasty flavors with ingredients full of nutrients.

This plan offers you energizing breakfasts and hearty dinners, all while introducing you to a diet that's kind to your heart, without compromising on taste or diversity. Prepare to dive into a week's worth of meals that are delicious and heart-healthy.

To create a 7-day meal plan that benefits heart health, it's crucial to choose dishes high in omega-3 fatty acids, fiber, lean proteins, and assorted fruits and vegetables while reducing intake of saturated fats and sugars. Below is a sample meal plan using your provided recipes, designed for balanced nutrition and variety each day.

Day 1

Breakfast: Energizing Oatmeal

Lunch: Quinoa-Based Oriental Salad

Dinner: Baked Salmon with a side of Stir Fry Broccoli, Onions, and Carrots

Snack: Green and Berry Smoothie

Day 2

Breakfast: Apple Cinnamon Smash Oatmeal

Lunch: Chicken Breast Delight with Grenade Salad

Dinner: Trout Scrambler served with Arugula and Mushroom Salad

Snack: Cheddar Turkey Deviled Egg

Day 3

Breakfast: Berry Blast Oats

Lunch: Cyprian Cheese and Greens Salad with Pesto Dressing

Dinner: Hot, Hot, Hot Salmon with Roasted Veggies

Snack: Toasted Almond Banana Mix

Day 4

Breakfast: Berry Blast English Muffin

Lunch: Heart Helping Cobb

Dinner: Turkish Meatballs in Marinara served with Broccoli-Kale with Avocado Toppings Rice Bowl

Snack: Spinach and Kale Blend

Day 5

Breakfast: Banana Bread

Lunch: Hearty Chicken Salad with Pasta

Dinner: Pepper Ginger Beef Stir-Fry with Mixed Vegetable Roast with Lemon Zest

Snack: Almond Surf Smoothie

Day 6

Breakfast: Energy Boost Smoothie

Lunch: Sun Crust Turkey Cuts with Butternut Squash with Turmeric Soup

Dinner: Grilled Eggplant served with Veggie Fried Rice

Snack: Go Green Blueberries

Day 7

Breakfast: Shrimp and Egg Fried Rice

Lunch: Salmon and Asparagus

Dinner: Mixed Vegetable Roast with Lemon Zest and a side of Apple and Onion Mix

Snack: Berry Blast Oats

This meal plan is designed to provide variety and balance, incorporating ingredients known for their heart-healthy benefits. Drinking plenty of water throughout the day and engaging in regular physical activity will further support heart health. Remember, it's always best to consult with a healthcare provider before starting any new diet, especially for individuals with specific health conditions like heart disease.

Recipe List

The recipes provided below serve as ideal examples of dishes that align with the principles of the cardiac diet, each thoughtfully integrated into the earlier shared meal plan to demonstrate what constitutes a heart-healthy meal.

Feel free to get creative with substitutions or alternative cooking methods for these dishes, ensuring you stay within the guidelines of the cardiac diet. Should you have any uncertainties, refer back to the cardiac diet food pyramid and the tips and suggestions outlined in the previous chapters to guide your choices.

Apple and Onion Mix

Ingredients:

- 1 medium-sized Granny Smith apple, finely diced
- 1/4 cup red onion, finely chopped
- 1/4 cup walnuts, toasted, finely chopped
- 1 tbsp. extra-virgin olive oil or walnut oil
- 1 tsp. lemon juice
- 1 tsp. honey
- 1/2 teaspoon sage, finely chopped
- a pinch of salt

Instructions:

1. Place apple dice, chopped onion, chopped walnuts, chopped sage, oil, honey, and lemon juice in a bowl.
2. Toss until all ingredients are evenly distributed and coated with honey-lemon dressing.
3. Sprinkle it with salt to taste.
4. Serve immediately.

Shrimp and Egg Fried Rice

Ingredients:

- 3/4 cup long-grain jasmine rice washed
- 1/2 cup water
- 1 cup chicken broth, no salt
- 4 oz. large shrimp
- 2 large eggs, beaten
- 2 cups sugar snap peas, trimmed and cut into two
- 1 cup shiitake mushrooms, caps only
- 1 cup carrots, diced into 1/4-inch bits
- 2 tbsp. low-sodium soy sauce
- 1 tbsp. garlic, minced
- 1 tbsp. fresh ginger, minced
- 1/4 tsp. red chili pepper, crushed
- 2 tbsp. vegetable oil
- 1/8 tsp. ground white pepper

Instructions:

1. Combine and boil the chicken broth and water in a small saucepan.
2. Add washed jasmine rice.
3. Reduce the heat to low.
4. Cover the saucepan with its lid.
5. Simmer until the rice has become tender, and the liquid has vaporized.
6. Remove from heat.

7. In a frying pan, heat the vegetable oil for half a minute.
8. Add minced garlic, minced ginger, and crushed red chili peppers.
9. Stir fry using a metal spatula for about 10 seconds, or until the mixture has become fragrant.
10. Add diced carrots and mushroom caps.
11. Stir fry for about 1 minute.
12. Add shrimp slices.
13. Stir fry for another minute.
14. Add sugar snap pear halves.
15. Stir fry for a minute, or until peas have turned bright green.
16. Remove from heat.
17. Add beaten eggs, cooked rice, soy sauce, and pepper.
18. While still off the heat, stir fry for about a minute or two, or until the shrimp are cooked through and the eggs have set.
19. Transfer into a bowl and serve while it is still hot.

Yield: 2 to 3 servings

Grilled Eggplant

Ingredients:

- 2 small eggplants or 1 large eggplant, around 1-1/4 to 1-1/12 lb. in total, sliced into half-inch-thick rounds
- 2 tbsp. extra-virgin olive oil
- salt

Instructions:

1. Preheat the grill using the medium-high setting.
2. Toss eggplant slices and olive oil in a bowl.
3. Sprinkle it with salt to taste.
4. Toss ingredients again.
5. Place eggplant slices onto the grill.
6. Turn over to the other side after about 4 minutes, or until charred spots have appeared on the underside.
7. Continue grilling until eggplant slices have become tender.
8. When storing, place it into an airtight container once it has cooled down, and then refrigerate.
9. Grilled eggplant can last for up to 4 days in a chilled condition.

Yield: 2 servings

Mixed Vegetable Roast with Lemon Zest

Ingredients:

- 1-1/2 cups broccoli florets
- 1-1/2 cups cauliflower florets
- 3/4 cup red bell pepper, diced
- 3/4 cup zucchini, diced
- 2 thinly sliced cloves of garlic
- 2 tsp. lemon zest
- 1 tbsp. olive oil
- a pinch of salt
- 1 tsp. dried and crushed oregano

Instructions:

1. Preheat the oven to 425°F for 25 minutes.
2. Combine garlic and florets of broccoli and cauliflower in a baking pan.
3. Drizzle oil evenly over the vegetables. Season with salt and oregano.
4. Stir the vegetables to coat them evenly.
5. Place the pan inside the oven and roast for 10 minutes.
6. Add zucchini and bell pepper to the mix. Toss to combine.

7. Continue roasting for 10 to 15 minutes more until the vegetables turn light brown.
8. Drizzle lemon zest over vegetables and toss.
9. Serve and enjoy.

Yield: 1 to 2 servings

Pepper Ginger Beef Stir-Fry

Ingredients:

- 6 oz. (175g) lean rump OR filet steak, thinly cut into strips across the grain
- 2 oz. (55g) mange tout trimmed
- 4 spring onions, chopped
- 1 small red bell pepper, deseeded and thinly cut into strips
- 1 small green or yellow bell pepper, deseeded and thinly cut into strips
- 1-1/2 tsp. Sichuan pepper, crushed
- 1 fresh red chili, deseeded and finely chopped
- 1 carrot, cut into thin sticks
- 0.8-inch (2 cm) fresh ginger, peeled and thinly cut into strips
- 1 clove garlic, finely chopped
- 1 tbsp. low-sodium soy sauce
- 4 tbsp. water
- 2-3 tsp. sunflower oil
- 1 tsp. cornflour
- 1 tsp. soft dark brown sugar

Instruction:

1. Mix cornflour and water in a small bowl until the texture has become smooth.

2. Stir in soy sauce and sugar until the particles have been completely dissolved. Set aside.
3. In a non-stick wok, heat 1 teaspoon of sunflower oil using the medium setting of the stove.
4. Add the beef strips and crushed pepper.
5. Stir-fry for about 3 to 4 minutes, or until the beef strips have turned brown.
6. Transfer the beef strips to a plate using a slotted spoon. Set aside.
7. Pour the remaining sunflower oil into the work.
8. Heat the oil using the medium setting.
9. Add the garlic, red chili, mange tout, peppers, carrot, spring onions, and ginger into the wok.
10. Stir-fry for 3 to 5 minutes or until the preferred texture is achieved.
11. Return the stir-fried beef strips from earlier.
12. Pour the cornflour mixture into the can.
13. Stir fry for 1 to 2 minutes, or until beef strips have become hot again.
14. Serve immediately over cooked rice or rice noodles.

Yield: 2 to 3 servings

Tip: If you are allergic to gluten, feel free to replace the low-sodium soy sauce used in this recipe with any gluten-free alternative.

Salmon and Asparagus

Ingredients:

- 2 salmon filets
- 14-oz. young potatoes
- 8 asparagus spears, trimmed and halved
- 2 handfuls cherry tomatoes
- 1 handful basil leaves
- 2 tbsp. extra-virgin olive oil
- 1 tbsp. balsamic vinegar

Instructions:

1. Heat oven to 428°F.
2. Arrange potatoes into a baking dish.
3. Drizzle potatoes with extra-virgin olive oil.
4. Roast potatoes until they have turned golden brown.
5. Place asparagus into the baking dish together with the potatoes.
6. Roast in the oven for 15 minutes.
7. Arrange cherry tomatoes and salmon among the vegetables.
8. Drizzle with balsamic vinegar and the remaining olive oil.
9. Roast until the salmon is cooked.

10. Throw in basil leaves before transferring everything to a serving dish.
11. Serve while hot.

Yield: 2 servings

Baked Salmon

Ingredients:

- 2 salmon filets
- 6 cups of fresh spinach
- 2 tsp. coconut oil
- 1/4 tsp. garlic powder
- 1/4 tsp. turmeric
- 3 large cloves of garlic
- lemon juice
- salt
- pepper

Instructions:

1. Preheat the oven to 400°F.
2. Line a baking dish with parchment paper.
3. Marinate salmon filets in lemon juice, coconut oil, garlic powder, turmeric, salt, and pepper.
4. Let it sit for a few minutes. This may also be done the night before to help the juices and flavor get into the salmon.
5. Once the oven is ready, bake the salmon for 15 minutes.
6. Cook some of the garlic in a pan with coconut oil.

7. Add spinach and cook until ready. Season with salt and pepper to taste.
8. Take salmon out of the oven and put spinach beside it.
9. Serve and enjoy.

Roasted Veggies

Ingredients:

- 1/2 lb. turnips
- 1/2 lb. carrots
- 1/2 lb. parsnips
- 2 shallots, peeled
- 1/4 tsp. ground black pepper
- 1 tbsp. extra-virgin olive oil
- 6 cloves garlic
- 3/4 tsp. kosher salt
- 2 tbsp. fresh rosemary needles

Instructions:

1. First, cut vegetables into bite-sized pieces.
2. Set the oven to 400°F.
3. Mix all the ingredients in a baking dish.
4. Roast the vegetables for 25 minutes until brown and tender.
5. Toss and roast again for 20–25 minutes.
6. Serve and enjoy while hot.

Trout Scrambler

Ingredients:

- 1 small potato, cut into 8 wedges
- 1/2 tsp. extra-virgin olive oil
- freshly ground black pepper, to taste
- 1 cup spinach
- 1 egg, scrambled
- 3 oz. trout filet
- dash of salt

Instructions:

1. Preheat the oven to 375°F.
2. Toss potatoes, 1/8 tsp. olive oil, and black pepper on a sheet tray.
3. Bake until the potatoes are tender, approximately 10 minutes.
4. Remove from the oven, toss in spinach, and set aside.
5. Heat 2 heavy-bottomed skillets over low heat.
6. In a small bowl, combine the egg and black pepper.
7. Put 1/8 tsp. olive oil in one pan, pour in the egg. Cook while stirring constantly until it reaches your desired doneness.
8. Place 1/8 tsp. olive oil in the second pan. Cook the fish until lightly browned for approximately 3 minutes.
9. Flip and cook until the fish are just beginning to flake but the center is still translucent, for about 2 minutes.

10. Serve the spinach and potato mixture with the scrambled egg and fish.
11. Just before eating, season the eggs and fish with a dash of salt.

Mixed Veggie Fried Rice

Ingredients:

- 2 tbsp. of minced garlic
- 2 eggs, beaten
- 1/4 cup of minced carrots and onions
- 1/2 cup of chopped tomatoes
- 1/8 cup of chopped parsley
- a cup of brown rice
- 1/4 tsp. of white ground pepper
- 1/4 tsp. salt
- 1/8 tsp. of ground turmeric for added flavor

Instructions:

1. Cook the rice and eggs separately.
2. Once you have cooked the eggs, slice them into thin strips. Pour olive or canola oil into the skillet.
3. Toss in the cooked brown rice.
4. Add the rest of the ingredients.
5. Sprinkle ground turmeric.
6. Add half a tsp. of balsamic vinegar, if desired.
7. Serve and enjoy.

Arugula and Mushroom Salad

Ingredients:

- 5 oz. arugula washed
- 1 lb. fresh mushrooms
- 1/4 tsp. shoyu
- 1/2 red onion
- 1 tbsp. olive oil
- 1 tbsp. mirin

For tofu cheese:

- 1/8 cup umeboshi vinegar
- 1/2 firm tofu

Instructions:

1. In a bowl, add the rinsed tofu. Crumble and pour in vinegar.
2. In a separate bowl add shoyu, red onions, salt, olive oil, and mirin.
3. Mix to combine.
4. Add in the arugula and toss to combine with the dressing.
5. Serve and enjoy.

Cypriot Cheese and Greens Salad with Pesto Dressing

Ingredients:

Salad:

- 2 heads of lettuce
- 1/4 bulb fennel
- 2 cucumbers
- 1 avocado
- 1/4 cup toasted almonds
- 1 packet halloumi/vegan cheese
- 1/4 cup basil leaves
- 1/8 cup dill
- black peppercorns
- 2 tbsp. lemon juice
- olive oil

Pesto sauce:

- 1 cup toasted almonds
- 1 lemon
- 1/2 cup arugula
- 1 cup olive oil

Instructions:

1. To make the pesto sauce, put all the ingredients in a food processor. Blend to smoothen.
2. Season with lemon juice, pepper, and salt to taste.

3. Transfer to a small bowl.
4. For the salad, place the herbs and vegetables in a large salad bowl. Toss well.
5. In a pan, fry the halloumi until the sides become crunchy.
6. Serve salad greens and pesto sauce together, garnished with crunchy halloumi.

Macrobiotic Bowl Medley

Ingredients:

- 1/2 cup brown rice
- 3 cup chard, roughly chopped
- 1 cup squash, diced
- 1 cup broccoli florets
- 1 cup black beans, thoroughly rinsed and drained
- 1 oz. kombu
- 1/2 cup sauerkraut, chopped

Sauce:

- 2 tbsp. sesame tahini
- 2 tbsp. sodium tamari
- 1 clove garlic
- 1 tbsp. ginger
- 1 lime, juiced

Instructions:

1. Boil 1 cup of water.
2. Add rice and allow it to boil. Cover and reduce heat and simmer for 40 minutes.
3. Remove from heat and allow to sit covered for another 10 minutes, then fluff with a fork.
4. Place beans in a pot with a kombu. Cover with water, and bring to a boil.

5. Reduce heat and simmer for 15-20 minutes. Drain and rinse after.
6. Place a steamer basket in a pot with water and bring to a boil.
7. Add broccoli, cover, and steam for 4-5 minutes then remove, keeping water in the pot.
8. Add squash, cover, and steam for 4-5 minutes then remove, keeping water in the pot.
9. Add chard, cover, and steam for 3-4 minutes, then remove.
10. Mix all the ingredients of the sauce.
11. Serve everything on a plate and enjoy!

Broccoli-Kale with Avocado Toppings Rice Bowl

Ingredients:

- 1/2 avocado
- 2 cups kale
- 1 cup broccoli florets
- 1/2 cup cooked brown rice
- 1 tsp. plum vinegar
- 2 tsp. tamari
- sea salt, to taste

Instructions:

1. In a small pot, simmer broccoli florets, and kale in about 3 tbsp. of water. Cook for 2 minutes.
2. Add tamari, vinegar, and cooked brown rice. Stir to combine.
3. Transfer pot contents into a medium-sized bowl and top with sliced avocado; sprinkle a dash of sea salt to taste.
4. Serve immediately.

Stir-fry Broccoli, Onions, and Carrots

Ingredients:

- 1 tsp. light olive oil
- 1-1/2 cups onion
- 2 cups medium-sized carrots
- 6 cups medium-sized broccoli
- 2-1/2-inch broccoli florets
- 1/4 tsp. of sea salt
- 1/2 cup of water

Instructions:

1. In a pan, heat sesame oil to medium-high heat.
2. Sauté onions. Add in carrots, broccoli, florets, and then water.
3. Season with sea salt, and cover the pan to bring to a boil.
4. Lower the heat and bring it to a simmer for 5 minutes.
5. Pour some soy sauce if needed.

Optional:

1. Top some pasta or rice with stir-fried vegetables.
2. Substitute other vegetables with cabbage, cauliflower, or yellow squash.
3. For additional flavor, sauté 1 tbsp. minced ginger before adding carrots.

Banana Bread

Ingredients:

- 1 cup olive oil mayonnaise
- 2 eggs
- 4 medium ripe bananas, mashed
- 2 tsp. vanilla extract
- 2 cups unbleached all-purpose flour
- 1 cup whole wheat flour
- 3/4 cup Brown Xylitol
- 2 tsp. baking soda
- 2 tsp. sea salt
- 2 tsp. cinnamon
- 1 tsp. baking powder
- Optional: flax, nuts, wheat germ, or whey protein

Instructions:

1. Preheat the oven to 350°F.
2. In a large mixing bowl, mix in banana, mayonnaise, eggs, and vanilla extract.
3. Combine the remaining dry ingredients in a different container.
4. Combine both mixtures by adding the dry one to the wet mixture.
5. Stir in the optional ingredients if desired.
6. Place the batter into a couple of loaf pans. Make sure to grease the pans first.

7. Place in the oven for about 45 to 50 minutes.
8. Let stand for 10 minutes. Remove from pan to finish cooling.
9. Serve and enjoy.

Yield: 6 to 8 servings

Butternut Squash with Turmeric Soup

Ingredients:

- 1 medium-sized (2-1/2 lbs.) butternut squash, peeled and chopped into 1-inch pieces, reserve the seeds
- 2 medium carrots, cut into 1-inch pieces
- 2-1/4 tsp. turmeric powder
- 1 large onion, roughly chopped
- 2 tbsp. light coconut milk
- 1 tbsp. vegetable soup base OR 1 vegetable bouillon cube
- 2-1/2 tbsp. extra-virgin olive oil
- 2-1/2 tsp. ground black pepper

Instructions:

1. Heat 2 tablespoons of oil in a large Dutch oven (cast-iron pot) using medium heat.
2. Add the onion and cover the pot with its lid.
3. Cook, while stirring occasionally, until onions have become tender.
4. Mix the soup base or bouillon with 6 cups of boiling water.
5. Stir until all powder or cube has been dissolved.
6. Add the carrots, squash, 2 teaspoons of turmeric, and 1/2 teaspoon of ground black pepper into the pot.
7. Cook for 1 minute while stirring occasionally.
8. Pour the soup broth into the pot.

9. Bring to a boil before reducing the heat.
10. Simmer for 18 to 22 minutes, or until vegetables have become very tender.
11. Heat oven to 375°F (191°C).
12. Toss 1/4 cup of the reserved seeds with the remaining oil, 1/4 teaspoon turmeric, and 1/4 teaspoon black pepper.
13. Roast for about 9 to 11 minutes, or until seeds have become crispy and golden brown
14. Puree the soup using an immersion blender.
15. Sprinkle with toasted seeds on top, and swirl in the coconut milk.
16. Serve immediately.

Tip: If you do not have an immersion blender, you may opt for a regular blender instead. Just remember to divide the soup into batches to get the right texture.

Yield: 3 to 4 servings

Cheddar Turkey Deviled Egg

Ingredients:

- 6 large organic eggs
- 2 slices nitrate-free turkey bacon
- 1/4 cup low-fat cheddar cheese, shredded OR grated
- 3 tbsp. light mayonnaise
- 1 tsp. white wine vinegar
- 1/2 tsp. chives, chopped
- 1/8 tsp. ground black pepper
- 1/8 tsp. salt

Instructions:

1. Place the eggs in a large pot or saucepan.
2. Pour cold water into the pot or pan until the water is covering the eggs by 1-1/2 inches.
3. Bring the water to a boil over high heat.
4. Once it has boiled, remove it from the stove.
5. Cover and let it stand for 12 to 15 minutes.
6. When it has cooled down, peel off the egg's shells.
7. Fry the bacon slices using medium-high heat in a non-stick skillet until bacon slices have become crispy but not burnt.
8. Transfer fried bacon to paper towels to drain off the excess oil.
9. Once it has cooled down, break down the bacon into small bits. Set aside.

10. Cut the hard-boiled eggs into half, lengthwise.
11. Gently carve out the egg yolks into a medium-sized bowl.
12. Arrange the hollowed-out egg halves in a flat container.
13. Add the rest of the ingredients to the bowl with the yolk.
14. Stir well until the texture has become smooth.
15. Transfer the mixture into a piping bag or resealable bag with a trimmed corner.
16. Pipe the yolk mixture back into the egg halves.
17. Sprinkle each filled egg half with bacon bits.
18. Serve immediately or after it has been chilled for at least half an hour.

Yield: 3 to 4 servings

Go Green Blueberries

Ingredients:

- 2 cups chopped spinach
- 1/4 cup water
- 1/3 cup chopped carrot
- 1/2 cup blueberries
- 1/2 cup chopped cucumber
- 1/4 cup almond milk
- 4 ice cubes

Instructions:

1. Using a blender, mix the water and spinach.
2. Slowly turn up the speed until no solid particles are present.
3. After the mixture has homogenized, add the other ingredients.
4. Continue to increase speed until you reach the maximum speed for 30 seconds.
5. Serve chilled.

Yield: 2

Spinach and Kale Blend

Ingredients:

- 1 cup spinach
- 1 cup chopped kale
- 3/4 cup water
- 1/2 cup chopped cucumber
- 1 green apple
- 1 cup chopped papaya
- 1 tbsp. ground flaxseed

Instructions:

1. Using a blender, mix water, spinach, and kale. Increase speed until all solid particles are gone.
2. Add the rest of the ingredients. Resume blending until reaching the maximum speed.
3. Maintain the maximum speed for 30 seconds before serving.
4. Serve chilled.

Yield: 2

Energy Boost Smoothie

Ingredients:

- 1 large rib of celery
- 1 tablespoon parsley
- 3/4 cup water
- 1/2 cup chopped cooked beets
- 1 small orange, segmented
- 3/4 cup chopped carrot

Instructions:

1. Using a blender, mix the water, parsley, and celery. Increase speed until all solid particles are gone.
2. Add the rest of the ingredients. Resume blending until reaching the maximum speed.
3. Maintain the maximum speed for 30 seconds before serving.
4. Serve chilled.

Yield: 2

Green and Berry Smoothie

Ingredients:

- 2 cups spinach
- 2 large kale leaves
- 3/4 cup water
- 1 large frozen banana
- 1/2 cup frozen mango
- 1/2 cup frozen peach
- 1 tbsp. ground flaxseeds
- 1 tbsp. almond butter or peanut butter

Instructions:

1. Using a blender, mix water, spinach, and kale until all solid particles are gone.
2. Add the frozen banana, mango, peach, ground flaxseeds and almond butter or peanut butter.
3. Increase speed gradually until reaching maximum speed for 30 seconds.
4. Serve chilled.

Yield: 2

Almond Surf Smoothie

Ingredients:

- 1 large banana
- 1 tbsp. almond butter
- 1 cup almond milk
- 1/8 tsp. vanilla extract
- 1 tbsp. wheat germ
- 1/8 tsp. ground cinnamon
- 3–4 ice cubes

Instructions:

1. Using a blender, place all the ingredients and start blending.
2. Increase speed until you reach the intermediate speed setting.
3. Maintain speed for 30 seconds before serving.
4. Serve chilled.

Yield: 1

Toasted Almond Banana Mix

Ingredients:

- 2 slices whole-wheat bread
- 2 tbsp. almond butter
- 1 small banana
- 1/8 tsp. ground cinnamon

Instructions:

1. Toast the slices of whole-wheat bread until golden brown.
2. Spread almond butter on one side of each slice of toast.
3. Thinly slice the banana and place it on top of one slice of toast.
4. Sprinkle cinnamon over the bananas.
5. Place the other slice of toast on top to make a sandwich.
6. Serve immediately and enjoy this quick and easy almond butter and banana treat!

Yield: 1 sandwich

Berry Blast English Muffin

Ingredients:

- 1 English muffin, halved
- 1 tbsp. cream cheese
- 4 strawberries
- 1/2 cup blueberries

Instructions:

1. Begin by toasting the English muffin halves until slightly crispy.
2. Spread cream cheese on each half of the English muffin.
3. Cut strawberries into thin slices and place on top of one half of the English muffin.
4. Top with blueberries.
5. Place the other half of the English muffin on top to create a sandwich.
6. Serve immediately.

Berry Blast Oats

Ingredients:

- 1-1/2 cups plain almond milk
- 1 cup oats
- 3/4 cup mix of blueberries and blackberries
- 2 tbsp. toasted pecans

Instructions:

1. In a small saucepan, bring 1-1/2 cups of almond milk to a boil.
2. Add in 1 cup of oats and stir until fully combined.
3. Reduce heat to low and let simmer for 5 minutes.
4. Stir in the mix of blueberries and blackberries until evenly distributed throughout the oatmeal.
5. Remove from heat and let cool for a few minutes.
6. Top with toasted pecans before serving.

Enjoy this delicious and nutritious breakfast option!

Yield: 2 servings

Apple Cinnamon Smash Oatmeal

Ingredients:

- 1-1/2 cups plain almond milk
- 1 cup oats
- 1 large Granny Smith apple
- 1/4 tsp. ground cinnamon
- 2 tbsp. toasted walnut pieces

Instructions:

1. In a small saucepan, bring 1-1/2 cups of almond milk to a boil.
2. Add in 1 cup of oats and stir until fully combined.
3. Reduce heat to low and let simmer for 5 minutes.
4. While the oatmeal is cooking, peel and dice the Granny Smith apple into small pieces.
5. Add diced apple and ground cinnamon to the oatmeal and stir until well combined.
6. Let simmer for an additional 2-3 minutes.
7. Top with toasted walnut pieces before serving.

This warm and comforting breakfast option is perfect for chilly mornings!

Yield: 2 servings

Energizing Oatmeal

Ingredients:

- 1/4 cup water
- 1/4 cup milk
- 1/2 cup oats
- 4 egg whites
- 1/8 tsp. ground cinnamon
- 1/8 tsp. ground ginger
- 1/4 cup blueberries

Instructions:

1. In a small saucepan, bring 1/4 cup of water and 1/4 cup of milk to a boil.
2. Add 1/2 cup of oats and stir until fully combined.
3. Reduce heat to low and let simmer for 5 minutes.
4. While the oatmeal is cooking, whisk together the egg whites, ground cinnamon, and ground ginger in a separate bowl.
5. Pour the egg white mixture into the oatmeal and stir until fully combined.
6. Let simmer for an additional 2-3 minutes, stirring occasionally.
7. Serve topped with fresh blueberries for an extra burst of flavor and energy!

Yield: 1 serving

Quinoa-Based Oriental Salad

Ingredients:

- 2 cups uncooked quinoa
- 4 cups vegetable broth
- 1 cup edamame
- 1/4 cup chopped green onion
- 1 1/2 tsp. chopped fresh mint
- 1/2 cup chopped carrot
- 1/2 cup chopped red bell pepper
- 1/8 tsp. pepper flakes
- 1/2 tsp. grated orange zest
- 2 tbsp. chopped fresh Thai basil
- juice from half an orange
- 1 tsp. sesame seeds
- 1 tbsp. sesame oil
- 1 tbsp. olive oil
- 1/8 tsp. black pepper

Instructions:

1. Begin by rinsing 2 cups of uncooked quinoa in cold water.
2. In a saucepan, bring 4 cups of vegetable broth to a boil.
3. Add the quinoa to the boiling broth and let cook for 15-20 minutes or until all the liquid is absorbed.

4. In a separate pan, sauté chopped carrots, red bell pepper, and edamame until tender.
5. Combine the cooked quinoa and sautéed vegetables in a large mixing bowl.
6. Add chopped green onion, fresh mint, grated orange zest, pepper flakes, Thai basil, sesame seeds, orange juice, sesame oil, olive oil, and black pepper to the quinoa mixture and stir until well combined.
7. Serve the oriental quinoa salad as a side dish or add your choice of protein to make it a complete meal.

This salad can be served warm or chilled, making it a perfect option for lunch on the go or a light dinner option during warmer months.

Yield: 4 servings

Hearty Chicken Salad with Pasta

Ingredients:

- 8 oz. penne pasta
- 1 (6-oz.) chicken breast
- 1 cup seedless red grapes
- 1/4 cup walnut pieces
- 1 tbsp. red wine vinegar
- 1/2 cup chopped celery
- 1/2 cup Greek yogurt
- 1/2 tsp. black pepper
- 1/8 tsp. salt

Instructions:

1. Cook 8 oz. of penne pasta according to package instructions, then drain and set aside.
2. In a separate pan, cook 6 oz. of chicken breast until fully cooked and lightly browned.
3. Once cooled, chop the chicken into bite-sized pieces and set aside.
4. In a large mixing bowl, combine the cooked pasta, chopped chicken, 1 cup of seedless red grapes, 1/4 cup of walnut pieces, and 1/2 cup of chopped celery.
5. In a separate small bowl, whisk together 1 tbsp. of red wine vinegar, 1/2 cup of Greek yogurt, 1/2 tsp. of black pepper, and 1/8 tsp. of salt.

6. Pour the dressing over the pasta and chicken mixture, and toss until well combined.
7. Serve the hearty chicken salad immediately or chill in the refrigerator for at least 30 minutes before serving to allow flavors to meld together.

This salad can be served as a light lunch option or as a side dish with dinner.

For added flavor, try adding diced avocado or crumbled feta cheese to the salad before serving.

Yield: 2-3 servings

Heart Helping Cobb

Ingredients:

- 4 slices of turkey bacon
- 5 cups spinach
- 1 cup sliced cremini mushrooms
- 1/2 cup shredded carrot
- 1/2 cucumber
- 1/2 (15-oz.) can kidney beans
- 1 large avocado
- 1/3 cup crumbled blue cheese

Instructions:

1. In a skillet, cook 4 slices of turkey bacon until crispy, then set aside on paper towels to drain.
2. In a large mixing bowl, combine 5 cups of spinach, 1 cup of sliced cremini mushrooms, and 1/2 cup of shredded carrot.
3. Dice half of a cucumber and add it to the salad mixture.
4. Rinse and drain 1/2 a can of kidney beans, then add to the salad.
5. Cut a large avocado into cubes and add it to the salad as well.
6. Crumble 1/3 cup of blue cheese over the top of the salad.
7. Toss all ingredients together until evenly combined.

8. Serve immediately with the crispy turkey bacon on top or chill in the refrigerator for 30 minutes before serving.

This nutrient-rich salad is great as a light lunch or can be served as a side dish with dinner.

For added protein, try adding grilled chicken or shrimp to make it a heartier meal.

Yield: 2-3 servings

Grenade Salad

Ingredients:

- 4 cups arugula
- 1 large avocado
- 1/2 cup sliced fennel
- 1/2 cup sliced Anjou pears
- 1/4 cup pomegranate seeds

Instructions:

1. In a mixing bowl, combine 4 cups of arugula and 1/2 cup of sliced fennel.
2. Dice a large avocado and add it to the salad mixture.
3. Thinly slice 1/2 an Anjou pear and add it to the salad.
4. Sprinkle 1/4 cup of pomegranate seeds over the top of the salad.
5. Toss all ingredients together until evenly combined.
6. Serve immediately as a refreshing and vibrant side dish or starter.

This Grenade Salad is packed with antioxidants and nutrients, making it a perfect addition to any meal.

For added flavor and texture, try adding crumbled goat cheese or chopped walnuts.

This salad can also be made into a full meal by adding grilled chicken, salmon, or tofu for added protein.

Yield: 2-3 servings

Chicken Breast Delight

Ingredients:

- 1 tsp. dried oregano
- 1/2 tsp. rosemary
- 1/2 tsp. garlic powder
- 1/8 tsp. salt
- finely ground black pepper
- 4 chicken breasts

Instructions:

1. Preheat your oven to 375°F.
2. In a small bowl, mix together 1 tsp. dried oregano, 1/2 tsp. rosemary, 1/2 tsp. garlic powder, and 1/8 tsp. salt.
3. Season both sides of the 4 chicken breasts with the herb mixture and black pepper.
4. Place the chicken breasts on a baking sheet and bake in the preheated oven for 25 minutes, or until cooked through.
5. Serve with your choice of sides such as roasted vegetables, quinoa, or a salad.

Yield: 4 servings

Sun Crust Turkey Cuts

Ingredients:

- 2 turkey breasts, cut into 1/4-inch thick slices
- 1-1/2 cups sunflower seeds
- 1/4 tsp. ground cumin
- 2 tbsp. chopped parsley
- 1/4 tsp. paprika
- 1/4 tsp. cayenne pepper
- 1/4 tsp. black pepper
- 1/3 cup whole wheat flour
- 3 egg whites

Instructions:

1. Preheat the oven to around 395 °F.
2. Mix the parsley, paprika, cumin, cayenne, sunflower seeds, and pepper in a processor.
3. Prepare the whites and flour in a separate container each.
4. Coat each breast part with the mixtures separately. Start with the flour mixture, followed by the whites, and then the processed mixture.
5. After coating all the breasts, prepare the pan.
6. Bake the breasts for approximately 12 minutes in the oven.

7. Flip each side and resume baking for another 12 minutes.
8. Serve hot.

Yield: 4 servings

Turkish Meatballs in Marinara

Ingredients:

- 1 lb. ground turkey
- 1/2 small onion
- 2 large cloves garlic,
- 1/4 cup red bell pepper
- 3 tbsp. chopped parsley
- 1/2 tsp. pepper flakes
- 1/8 tsp. ground cumin
- 1/2 tsp. dried pre-mixed Italian herbs
- 1/8 tsp. black pepper
- 1 egg
- 1/4 cup breadcrumbs
- 1/8 tsp. salt
- 4 tbsp. olive oil
- 1 (16-oz.) jar marinara sauce
- 1/2 cup feta cheese

Instructions:

1. Preheat the oven to 375°F.
2. In a mixing bowl, combine the ground turkey, chopped onion, minced garlic, diced red bell pepper, chopped parsley, pepper flakes, cumin, Italian herbs and black pepper.
3. Add in the egg and breadcrumbs to the mixture and mix well.

4. Shape into small meatballs using your hands or a scoop.
5. Heat the olive oil in a skillet over medium heat.
6. Add the meatballs to the skillet and cook until browned on all sides, around 8 minutes.
7. Remove the meatballs from the skillet and place them in an oven-safe dish.
8. Pour marinara sauce over the meatballs and sprinkle with feta cheese on top.
9. Bake in the oven for 15-20 minutes until the cheese is melted and bubbly.
10. Serve hot with your choice of side dishes, such as pasta or rice.

Yield: 16 meatballs

Hot, Hot, Hot Salmon

Ingredients:

- 2 tsp. chili powder
- 1 tsp. ground cumin
- 1 tsp. molasses
- 1/8 tsp. salt
- 1/8 tsp. black pepper
- 4 (4-oz.) salmon filets
- 1/2 orange, juice only
- 2 tbsp. olive oil

Instructions:

1. Preheat the oven to 425°F.
2. In a small bowl, mix together the chili powder, cumin, molasses, salt, and black pepper.
3. Rub the spice mixture all over the salmon filets.
4. In another bowl, mix the orange juice and olive oil.
5. Place the seasoned salmon filets in an oven-safe dish and pour the orange juice mixture over them.
6. Bake for 12-15 minutes, until the salmon is cooked through and flakes easily with a fork.
7. Serve hot with your choice of side dishes, such as roasted vegetables or quinoa.

Yield: 4 servings

Taste of Mediterranean

Ingredients:

- 1 cup uncooked couscous
- 1 1/4 cups water
- 1 (16-oz.) can artichoke hearts
- 1/2 cup kalamata olives
- 1 (12-oz.) jar roasted red pepper
- 1/2 cup feta cheese
- 1 cup cherry tomatoes
- 1/2 small onion
- 1/4 tsp. chopped oregano
- 1/4 tsp. chopped fresh mint
- 1/2 tsp. Pepper flakes
- 4 tbsp. extra virgin olive oil
- Lemon Juice from a Single Lemon
- a piece of black pepper

Instructions:

1. Cook couscous according to package instructions, using water instead of broth for a lighter dish.
2. Drain and chop artichoke hearts and roasted red pepper into bite-sized pieces.
3. Slice kalamata olives in half and cut cherry tomatoes in quarters.
4. Finely dice the onion and chop oregano and mint leaves.

5. In a large bowl, combine the cooked couscous, artichoke hearts, kalamata olives, roasted red pepper, feta cheese, cherry tomatoes, onion, oregano, and mint.
6. Drizzle with extra virgin olive oil and lemon juice.
7. Add a pinch of black pepper and red pepper flakes for an extra kick.
8. Toss all the ingredients together until well combined.
9. Serve as a side dish or add grilled chicken or shrimp for a complete meal.

Enjoy the taste of the Mediterranean with this refreshing and flavorful couscous salad!

Yield: 4 servings

Avocado and Tomato Whole Wheat Pasta Salad

Ingredients:

- 2 cups whole wheat pasta (cooked and cooled)
- 1 ripe avocado, diced
- 1 cup cherry tomatoes, halved
- 1/4 cup red onion, finely chopped
- 2 tablespoons extra virgin olive oil
- 1 tablespoon balsamic vinegar
- Salt and pepper to taste
- Fresh basil leaves for garnish

Instructions:

1. In a large bowl, combine the cooked and cooled whole wheat pasta with diced avocado, halved cherry tomatoes, and finely chopped red onion.
2. Drizzle with extra virgin olive oil and balsamic vinegar.
3. Season with salt and pepper to taste.
4. Toss all the ingredients together until well combined.
5. Garnish with fresh basil leaves.
6. Serve as a light and refreshing lunch or dinner option.

This avocado and tomato whole wheat pasta salad is packed with healthy fats, fiber, and nutrients for a satisfying and nutritious meal!

Lentil Vegetable Soup

Ingredients:

- 1 tablespoon olive oil
- 1 onion, chopped
- 2 carrots, diced
- 2 stalks celery, diced
- 2 cloves garlic, minced
- 1 cup dried lentils, rinsed
- 4 cups low-sodium vegetable broth
- 1 can diced tomatoes (no salt added)
- 1 teaspoon thyme
- Salt and pepper to taste
- 2 cups spinach leaves

Instructions:

1. In a large pot, heat olive oil over medium heat.
2. Add onion, carrots, celery, and garlic. Cook until vegetables are softened.
3. Stir in dried lentils and vegetable broth.
4. Bring to a boil, then reduce heat and let simmer for 20 minutes.
5. Add diced tomatoes and thyme to the pot.
6. Season with salt and pepper to taste.
7. Let simmer for an additional 10 minutes.

8. Add spinach leaves and cook until wilted.
9. Serve hot and enjoy the hearty flavors of this lentil vegetable soup!

Grilled Vegetable and Hummus Wrap

Ingredients:

- Whole wheat tortillas
- 1 zucchini, sliced lengthwise
- 1 bell pepper, sliced
- 1 tablespoon olive oil
- Salt and pepper to taste
- 1/2 cup hummus
- Mixed greens or spinach leaves

Instructions:

1. Preheat a grill or grill pan over medium-high heat.
2. Brush the zucchini and bell pepper slices with olive oil, then season with salt and pepper.
3. Grill the vegetables for about 5 minutes on each side, until slightly charred and tender.
4. Warm the tortillas in a separate pan or in the microwave.
5. Spread about 2 tablespoons of hummus on each tortilla, leaving an inch border around the edges.
6. Top with grilled vegetables and a handful of mixed greens or spinach leaves.
7. Roll up the tortillas tightly, tucking in the ends as you go.
8. Cut in half diagonally and serve.

Apple Cinnamon Oatmeal

Ingredients:

- 1 cup rolled oats
- 2 cups almond milk
- 1 apple, diced
- 1 teaspoon cinnamon
- 1 tablespoon maple syrup (optional)
- Chopped nuts for topping (walnuts or almonds)

Instructions:

1. In a medium saucepan, bring the almond milk to a boil.
2. Stir in the rolled oats, diced apple, and cinnamon.
3. Reduce heat to low and let simmer for 10-15 minutes, stirring occasionally.
4. If desired, stir in maple syrup for added sweetness.
5. Serve hot and top with chopped nuts for added crunch.
6. Enjoy this cozy and delicious breakfast on a chilly morning!

Turkey and Veggie Stuffed Peppers

Ingredients:

- 4 bell peppers, halved and seeds removed
- 1 tablespoon olive oil
- 1 pound ground turkey
- 1 onion, chopped
- 2 cloves garlic, minced
- 1 zucchini, diced
- 1 cup cooked quinoa
- 1 can diced tomatoes (drained)
- 1 teaspoon Italian seasoning
- Salt and pepper to taste
- Shredded low-fat mozzarella cheese (optional)

Instructions:

1. Preheat the oven to 375°F (190°C). Place the bell pepper halves in a baking dish.
2. Heat olive oil in a skillet over medium heat. Add ground turkey, onion, and garlic. Cook until the turkey is browned.
3. Stir in the zucchini, cooked quinoa, diced tomatoes, and Italian seasoning. Season with salt and pepper.
4. Spoon the turkey and veggie mixture into the bell pepper halves.

5. Bake for about 25-30 minutes, or until the peppers are tender.
6. Top with shredded mozzarella cheese during the last 5 minutes of baking if desired.

Conclusion

Congratulations on reaching the conclusion of our Heart Disease Recipes Guide! This is a significant milestone in your health and wellness journey, and you should feel proud of the commitment you've made to nurture your heart through mindful nutrition. By choosing to explore and integrate these recipes into your daily life, you've taken a powerful step towards supporting your heart health and overall well-being.

First and foremost, we want to extend our sincerest thanks to you for engaging with this guide. It's an honor to have been part of your quest for heart-healthy culinary options, and we commend your dedication to making positive dietary changes. Your willingness to adapt and incorporate new, nutritious recipes into your meals is a testament to your commitment to living a healthier life.

Throughout this guide, we've navigated a variety of recipes, each carefully curated to cater to the needs of those looking to enhance their heart health through diet. From the invigorating flavors of our morning smoothies to the rich, satisfying textures of our wholesome dinners, every recipe was designed with both your palate and your heart in mind. These dishes are not just meals; they are stepping stones towards a heart-healthy lifestyle that doesn't compromise on taste or satisfaction.

One crucial insight we hope you've gained from this guide is the understanding that heart-healthy eating can be both delicious and diverse. The notion that diets catered towards improving heart health are bland or restrictive is a myth we aimed to dispel. With the right ingredients and a bit of creativity, you can enjoy a wide array of flavorful, nutritious meals that nourish your heart and delight your taste buds.

Adopting a heart-healthy diet is about making informed, mindful choices. It's about recognizing the power of food as medicine and understanding how certain ingredients can positively impact your heart health. Omega-3 fatty acids, whole grains, lean proteins, and a bounty of fruits and vegetables have all played starring roles in our recipes, showcasing the variety and richness of heart-healthy eating.

We encourage you to view this guide not as an endpoint but as a beginning. The path to heart health is ongoing, and there are always new recipes to try, ingredients to discover, and dietary habits to explore. Keep experimenting with the recipes from this guide, adjusting them to your tastes and dietary needs. Remember, the goal is to find joy and satisfaction in heart-healthy eating, creating a sustainable lifestyle that you look forward to each day.

Beyond diet, we hope this guide has inspired you to consider other aspects of heart health, such as regular exercise, stress management, and avoiding harmful habits like smoking and excessive drinking. A holistic approach to heart health, incorporating both dietary and lifestyle changes, is key to achieving and maintaining optimal heart function.

Your engagement with this guide is a powerful reminder of your agency in your health journey. You've shown that you're not waiting passively for health improvements—you're actively pursuing a better, healthier life. We applaud your initiative and encourage you to continue with this proactive mindset.

Thank you once again for joining us on this culinary adventure. It's been a privilege to share these recipes and insights with you, and we hope they've provided you with valuable tools for your heart health toolkit. Remember, every meal is an opportunity to nourish your heart, and with each heart-healthy choice, you're taking a step towards a brighter, healthier future.

Keep exploring, keep learning, and most importantly, keep enjoying the process. Your heart health journey is uniquely yours, and there's so much beauty in the path you're carving for yourself. Here's to your continued health and happiness, and many more delicious, heart-friendly meals ahead.

FAQ

What are the best foods to eat for heart health?

The best foods for heart health include fruits and vegetables, whole grains, lean proteins (such as fish rich in omega-3 fatty acids, poultry, and plant-based proteins), low-fat or non-fat dairy, and healthy fats (like those found in avocados, nuts, seeds, and olive oil). Incorporating a variety of these foods into your diet can help maintain a healthy heart.

Are there foods I should avoid if I have heart disease?

Yes, it's advisable to limit or avoid foods high in saturated and trans fats, excessive salt (sodium), added sugars, and processed foods. These include deep-fried foods, processed meats (like sausages and bacon), full-fat dairy products, sugary beverages (including soda and juice with added sugar), and packaged snacks high in sodium.

How does fiber benefit heart health?

Fiber benefits heart health by helping to lower levels of bad cholesterol (LDL) in the blood, which can reduce the risk of heart disease. Soluble fiber, in particular, found in foods like oats, beans, lentils, apples, and flaxseeds, is effective in lowering cholesterol levels. Fiber also helps in weight management and maintains digestive health, contributing to overall heart health.

Can I still eat red meat if I'm on a heart disease diet?

While you don't have to eliminate red meat, it's important to choose lean cuts and limit your intake to a few times a month. Opt for smaller portions and consider it more as a side dish rather than the main component of your meal. Alternatives like fish, poultry, and plant-based proteins are preferable for regular consumption.

Is it okay to drink alcohol when following a heart disease diet?

Moderation is key when it comes to alcohol. Some studies suggest that small amounts of certain types of alcohol, like red wine, may have heart benefits. However, excessive alcohol consumption can lead to increased blood pressure, heart failure, and obesity, negating any potential benefits. It's best to consult with your healthcare provider for personalized advice.

How does salt intake affect heart disease?

High salt intake is linked to increased blood pressure, a major risk factor for heart disease. Reducing salt in your diet can help lower blood pressure and decrease the risk of heart disease and stroke. Aim to consume less than 2,300 milligrams of sodium per day, and be mindful of hidden salts in processed and restaurant foods.

Can lifestyle changes alone manage heart disease, or is medication always necessary?

Lifestyle changes, such as a heart-healthy diet, regular physical activity, managing stress, and not smoking, play a crucial role in managing heart disease and can sometimes be enough to control mild conditions. However, depending on the severity of the heart disease, medications or other medical interventions may be necessary. Always work closely with your healthcare provider to determine the best treatment plan for you.

References and Helpful Links

Heart disease - Symptoms and causes - Mayo Clinic. (2022, August 25). Mayo Clinic. https://www.mayoclinic.org/diseases-conditions/heart-disease/symptoms-causes/syc-20353118

What is Cardiovascular Disease? (2024, January 10). www.heart.org. https://www.heart.org/en/health-topics/consumer-healthcare/what-is-cardiovascular-disease

Strategies to prevent heart disease. (2023, August 17). Mayo Clinic. https://www.mayoclinic.org/diseases-conditions/heart-disease/in-depth/heart-disease-prevention/art-20046502

Restivo, J. (2023, November 9). Heart-healthy foods: What to eat and what to avoid. Harvard Health. https://www.health.harvard.edu/heart-health/heart-healthy-foods-what-to-eat-and-what-to-avoid

Foods that are bad for your heart. (n.d.). WebMD. https://www.webmd.com/heart-disease/ss/slideshow-foods-bad-heart

Rd, V. S. M. (2023, July 11). 7-Day Heart-Healthy Meal Plan: 1,200 calories. EatingWell. https://www.eatingwell.com/article/289245/7-day-heart-healthy-meal-plan-1200-calories/

Ldn, S. H. R. (2024, April 15). Heart-Healthy Diet Plan for Beginners. EatingWell. https://www.eatingwell.com/article/7884046/heart-healthy-diet-plan-for-beginners/

Heart-healthy recipes. (2023, November 7). https://www.mayoclinic.org/healthy-lifestyle/recipes/heart-healthy-recipes/rcs-20077163

Berry, E., & Franke, K. (2024, April 1). 59 Heart-Healthy recipes to make for an easy dinner tonight. Woman's Day. https://www.womansday.com/food-recipes/food-drinks/g2176/hearty-healthy-recipes/

www.ingramcontent.com/pod-product-compliance
Lightning Source LLC
LaVergne TN
LVHW012030060526
838201LV00061B/4545